MUSCULAR ARMS AND SHOULDERS

A BOSCO BOOK

AUTHORED BY
HARRY B. PASCHALL

Originally Published in 1953

PUBLISHED BY O'Faolain Patriot LLC,
Copyright 2012 info@PhysicalCultureBooks.com

Published in the United States of America

ISBN-13: 978-1477576120

ISBN-10: 1477576126

To Order More Copies Visit: Physical Culture
Books.com

and all responsibility and/or liabilities that might result from the uninformed or misinformed application of the techniques identified herein as well as for any unsupervised physical fitness training.

Finally, the publisher disclaims any and all liabilities arising from the use of any equipment featured in this book and makes no representations as to the utility, safety, or adequacy of the equipment generally or with respect to any specific purpose.

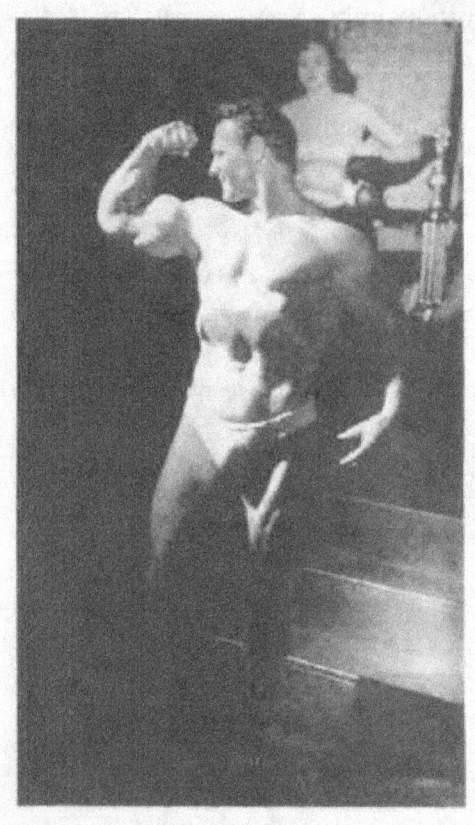

The Author respectfully dedicates this book on muscular arms and shoulders to the man who possesses the most perfect development in the world—JOHN C. GRIMEK.

CONTENTS

FOREWORD

I wish I could state boldly that this book is written by the "World's Foremost Authority on Physical Culture", but I am afraid to make such a categorical statement. After all, I have only been a student of body building and weight lifting for forty years. A lifetime is not long enough to learn all there is to know about this vital subject.

So I shall merely say that the contents of this book represent what one man has learned through close association with the leading men of muscle, through practical, realistic shoulder-to-shoulder workouts in the world's leading training centres. The impractical methods have been weeded out, and this brief work gives you the gist of accepted practice of the present-day stars. I believe firmly that anyone who puts this information to practical use will be able to develop strong, shapely and perfectly muscled arms and shoulders.

It may be of some small comfort to other muscleheads to know that the author is still as much in love with barbells and dumb-bells as he was forty years ago, and still uses them regularly and happily.

FLORIDA 1953.

HARRY B. PASCHALL

CHAPTER ONE

ARMS . . . AND THE MAN

ON THE beach at Cape May, several years ago, we watched a little incident so typical it might have occurred anywhere in the world. A family group was enjoying the salt surf and the sunshine, and papa was, like so many others, a camera fan. He trained the lens on each member of the family in turn, and finally focused on ten-year-old Junior. The youngster immediately assumed the arms-cocked-at-right-angles muscle pose familiar to Strongmen for generations, and tensed biceps almost as big as oysters. " Look at me, Pop," he shouted, " I'm Superman! "

It is so natural to think of the upper arms when one mentions the word " muscle ", that it must almost be instinctive. As kids in the school yard, we remember gathering around the most athletic schoolboy and asking him to " Let us feel your muscle We never thought of feeling the vastus externus, the lattissimus dorsi, or the pectoralis major—no siree, Bob—it was always the biceps. Powerfully developed arms remain, through the years, the hallmark of the strength champion, and it is logical that the average physical culturist devotes a great deal of thought and time to the culture of the arms.

The very first training book we bought as a fourteen- year-old boy was entitled Strong Arms and Shoulders. In forty years we have come full circle. Instead of reading about lumpy arms, we are writing about them ourselves, and we hope to show you that we have learned something of the subject in the ensuing four decades.

The most important single thing we have learned is that the deltoid muscles of the shoulders are really more worthy of consideration than the various muscles of the arm if you are aiming at an impressive physique. We will go even further—the shoulders are the KEY to masculine physical perfection.

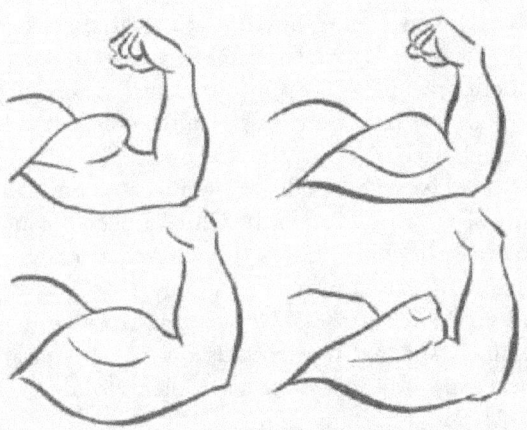

There are almost as many different types of arms as there are people! Some, as shown in the upper left, have a short biceps, with long tendon. The upper right picture shows the long, full biceps which crowds the joint. Lower left, comparative over-development of the triceps in relation to biceps. Lower right, the unique "lump on a lump" effect achieved by some musclemen through "cramp" curls.

Fortunately, it is impossible to develop the deltoid muscles to their full power and beauty without also exercising the arms thoroughly, so the possessor of broad, rounded, muscular shoulders is invariably fitted with well-developed arms as well. The opposite is also true; it is possible to build bulky arms without an appropriately large shoulder development—so it is important that the seeker of perfection approach the subject from the proper angle. Remember—shoulders first; arms second.

Let me tell you a little inside story, not generally known, which brings out the truth of the axiom above. Back in 1949, at the " Mr. USA " physique competition in California, among dozens of contestants, there were three outstanding, world-famous bodybuilders: John Grimek, Clancy Ross and Steve Reeves. The latter two were then at the zenith of their powers, and each had been strongly touted as possible winners. Reeves, as a matter of fact, in that year won the " Mr. Universe " award in London. When posing, under the spotlight, all three men showed tremendous muscular bulk and separation, and presented a problem to the very capable judges. The contest was decided very simply. Backstage the officials observed the men walking about in a relaxed condition—no strutting; no flexion. In repose the full roundness of the incomparable Grimek shoulders was so convincing that all doubt was instantly removed. The only serious question then rose: who would be rated second and who third? This is what caused the long discussion among the judges at that contest, which was commented upon at great length in some of the muscle magazines. Shoulders had won over biceps.

Nature can be trusted as the most efficient of all muscle "carpenters"; she always builds up the proper muscle structure when the body makes the right and natural demand. Well-rounded deltoids are not an accident; they emphasise arm development because of the shortening effect they give to the upper arm. The sweep of the Grimek deltoid adds much to the muscular bulk of his biceps. You simply cannot have a perfect arm unless the deltoid is developed too, because the shoulder is necessary to give Power to the arm. The best lifters are noted for shoulder development. You may say, at this point, " who cares about deltoids—what I want is an eighteen-inch biceps ". The point I would like to make is that an eighteen-inch arm (providing you can get it) without comparable deltoid development will not look as big as a sixteen-inch biceps which does have proper shoulder muscles to go with it.

In carefully considering the impressive points of the male physique, the average judge's eyes will start at the top. The breadth of the shoulders receives careful consideration before any other part of the body receives attention. In my own experience as a contest judge, I have eliminated many men from the competition at this very first glance because their deltoid development did not measure up to championship calibre. And, again, many other men who did not possess comparable development below the shoulders have been given a chance in the contest because of outstanding shoulders.

What do we look for in the perfect male physique? Certainly our first consideration must be given to that part of their muscular equipment which accentuates maleness. We do not look for the soft

11

curves of the female; we regard with horror the current tendency to over-development of the male pectoral muscles. We do not want broad hips. We look instinctively for wide shoulders; the V taper from armpits to waist; the swelling outward curve of the thighs and an adequate muscular calf development. And of all these things, powerful shoulders count first.

This little book is intended as a specialized treatise on the arms and shoulders, but we believe all specialization must be considered in the light of the whole physique; each part must be a harmonious portion of the whole. We might interject at this point a bit of advice to the serious bodybuilder. Your chances as a competitor will be greatly enhanced if you constantly check your standard against that of the officials who will judge you. If you have good development in three key places, you improve your position. These three parts are: the shoulders — the V taper formed by the latissimus dorsi of the back — and outstanding calf development. Three equally important drawbacks to the perfect physique should also be eliminated: Under-development of the deltoids in comparison with the arms — an unsightly over-development of both latissimus and pectorals (particularly the pectorals) — and ungainly thigh and hip development (particularly the sagging inner thigh muscles just above the knee).

Having now issued my official warning, after the manner of an arresting officer (" anything you say may be used against you "), let us return to the real meat of this volume—the development of the arms and shoulders. Can everybody secure an eighteen-inch arm? This depends largely upon the individual, for throughout the world there are no two men alike in their potentials. The small man has a smaller potential than the six-footer, naturally. Anyone under 5' 6" who develops sixteen- and-a-half-inch arms will look just as good as the six-footer who has 18". Yet many men around 5' 6" have developed eighteen-inch arms. We offer Roy Hilligenn (" Mr. America " 1951) as an example. John Grimek stands 5' 8|", and has full eighteen-inch arms. The largest shapely muscular arms of which we have record were those of Louis Uni (Apollon), who possessed twenty-inch biceps with matching deltoids. Our old training partner, John McWilliams, got his arms up to well over 20". McWilliams is a strong six feet, and Apollon stood about 6' 4". We would conclude that anybody with fair bone structure and leverage, who stands 5' 7" or taller, has a potential of eighteen-inch upper arms.

Structure has quite a bit to do with arm development. We have always thought that John Grimek had the ideal muscular leverage, and that this accident of birth gave him a great advantage in attaining his position as the best-developed man of his era. The length of the upper- arm bones in relation to those of the forearm, makes the difference between a good " natural " presser and a poor one. Further, the point of insertion of the biceps and brachialis in the bones of the forearm determines whether or not a man will be a " natural " curler. Actually, the poorer your leverage, the greater your potentialities for muscular development to compensate for it.

We have watched many new men come into the gymnasium and start on a standard course of barbell exercise. Some of these men grew like weeds in a garden; their biceps immediately took on shape and size, completely filling the upper arm with a ball-like lump of muscle. Others, using exactly the same exercise, failed to get such development. Why? The reason was the difference in arm leverage. We have also noticed that every individual arm has a slightly different shape. Some have full, thick biceps which crowd the joint, and others have a hump close to the shoulder and a long low space several inches in length at the insertion in the elbow. We have sketched some of these different types of arms for inclusion in this book. All anyone can do is to fully develop the type of arm which he naturally possesses.

We are constitutionally allergic to long, dry-as-dust, anatomical discussions about bones, muscles and sinews, but some simple understanding of the structure of the arms may help the student to more readily build up to his full potential. To that end, we have included a simple drawing of the arm in this book. The Biceps Brachii (hereinafter referred to by the simpler term of biceps) is a two-headed muscle (and in its highly developed state, you can see the division in the form of an indentation) with its origin in the bone of the shoulder, and its insertion in the radius bone of the forearm. This muscle does not, as many think, constitute the great bulk of the upper arm. It is possibly less useful as a muscle than the Brachialis Anticus, the muscle which goes into action when you lift a weight to the shoulder, and which forms the side of the upper arm. A great deal of your muscular bulk is represented by the brachialis when you double up your arm in the accepted right-angle position. When you do rowing movements, this muscle does the work. The largest muscle of the upper arm is the three-headed Triceps on the back of the arm, which is shaped like a horseshoe when the arm is straightened to the rear if the arm is fully developed. This muscle is much stronger than the biceps, and comes into use when weights are pressed over head, and in various other ways. To simplify: The biceps comes into play when you turn the palm of the hand from down to up, and assists when the brachialis " curls " or bends the arm to the shoulder. The triceps come into play when you straighten the arms. The supinator muscles of the forearm come into play when you grip an object and turn the hand inward; the pronator muscles when you turn the hand back upon the forearm, as in the reverse curling motion.

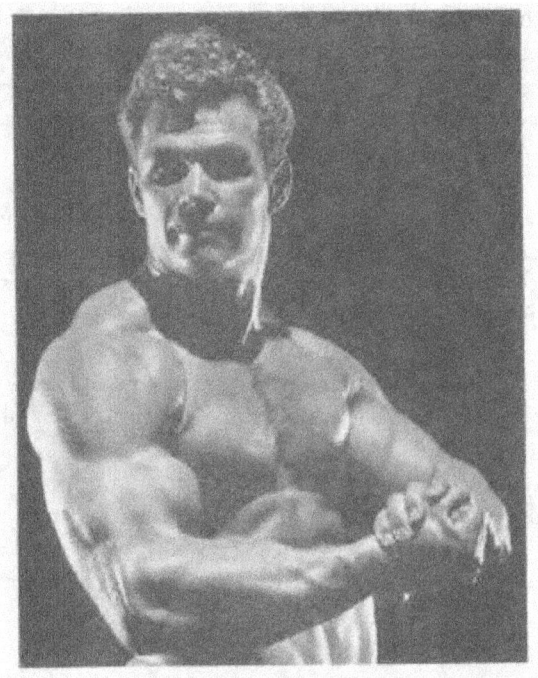

Roy Hilligenn, Mr. America, 1951, has one of the world's finest physiques. His 18 inch arms are in keeping with the balance of his tremendous musculature. He is just as strong as he looks, and agile as a panther.

Now let us turn to a consideration of ways and means to fully develop these muscles.

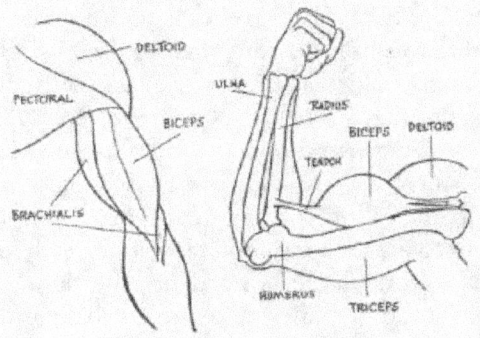

THE ANATOMY OF
THE ARM AND SHOULDER

DELTOID
PECTORAL
BICEPS
BRACHIALIS

ULNA
RADIUS
BICEPS
DELTOID
TENDON
HUMERUS
TRICEPS

17

CHAPTER TWO

A DISCUSSION OF TRAINING METHODS

AMONG ALL classes of athletes, nobody can deny that weightlifters have the best arms. Next to them, we would place handbalancers and roman ring performers. Some workmen get very capable arms in the performance of their regular tasks, notably men who use pick and shovel, the farmer, and men in various phases of the construction or building trades. We recall quite well our early days, when we worked with a building gang during our school vacation, eyeing the plasterers' bare arms as they worked at their craft. We noticed several of these men with extraordinary biceps, developed by the twisting and turning-in of the hand as they wielded their trowels and mortar boards. Among lumberjacks and farmers, we noted very-well-developed forearms and brachialis, due to sawing movements, while gripping hard with the hands. These men also built amazing hands and wrists, and were very strong.

We knew one man, many years ago, who worked in a factory, and used a spanner in a peculiar way for eight hours every day. He developed the large bulge of muscle of the forearm which bulks up when you hold the arm in the " gooseneck " position, so that his forearm was a full two inches larger than his upper arm at the biceps. His arm looked like a case of elephantitis, and was a revolting sight. The reason for this was, of course, that he had developed this one portion of the arm at the expense of all the other muscles, which were given practically no exercise at all. This fellow, incidentally, was almost unbeatable at the sport of wrist-turning, as was every other workman we have run across who devoted a lot of time to turning and twisting the arm while using a wrench or spanner in his daily work.

This man has remained in my memory over the years as a warning against over-specialization in exercise. You CAN overdevelop certain parts of the body at the expense of others, and you may lose athletic proportions in doing so. Some roman ring performers I have seen remind me of this chap, because they are all arms, shoulders, pectoral and latissimus muscles, with small legs. This is sometimes true of handbalancers as well, with the exception of the " bottom man ", who necessarily develops good legs in holding up the others. If you want almost ideal all-round development, tumblers, as a class, are unexcelled. An acrobat must develop almost every muscle in order to have muscular co-ordination and control sufficient to enable him to flip and leap and twist through the air in his amazing convolutions. The ideal weightlifter should be a tumbler as well.

My first course in arm exercise was quite simple. It employed almost exactly the same basic exercises you will find in many mail-order muscle courses to-day. First, the chinning exercise for the biceps. Second, the pushups for the triceps. The chins were done with the palms of the hands turned in, and we found that we got better results when we kept our hands quite wide apart. This was a personal matter, and many find they do better with hands close together. The push-ups were first done on the floor, then with feet elevated on the seat of a chair, and later we did pushups while in the handstand position with our heels against a wall for balance. We also did dips between two chairbacks, with our knees bent to keep from touching the floor.

Many of the first sixteen-inch biceps were created in this very way. We can recall Earle Liederman and Charles Atlas training at the YMCA in New York, doing innumerable routines or " sets " of dips between the parallel bars. This was all very well, but too many dips call upon the pectoral muscles for aid, particularly when the triceps tire, and men who do hundreds of these are apt to get an overdevelopment of the pectoral muscles.

Also, they do not get the proper deltoid musculature to fit in with their big arms. Many of our latter-day musclemen have carried this dipping even further by tying a weight to the feet. They, too, are trifling with disaster, because of over-emphasis on the breast muscles.

Boxers, who punch the light and heavy bag, have very good arms as a rule. It has often amazed me to find boxers with a splendid biceps development, when one would think most of their effort was devoted to straightening the arms in the punching motion, thus tending to develop the triceps. However, a little thought will explain this—a boxer twists his hand as he strikes, and this pronation of the hand from palm up to palm down is the very motion for which the biceps is designed. It would be well for you to remember this later on when we consider exercises for the biceps.

If you are to obtain the ultimate in arm and shoulder development, you are going to have to use progressive weight training. We have never known eighteen-inch arms developed in any other way. So it is necessary that we spend a little time in considering the best methods used by the current crop of muscle men. There are more eighteen-inch arms to-day than ever before in history, and it is a direct result of arm specialization with dumbbells and barbells. We have trained with many of these men, and may be able to save you time and energy by setting down what we believe to be the true essentials.

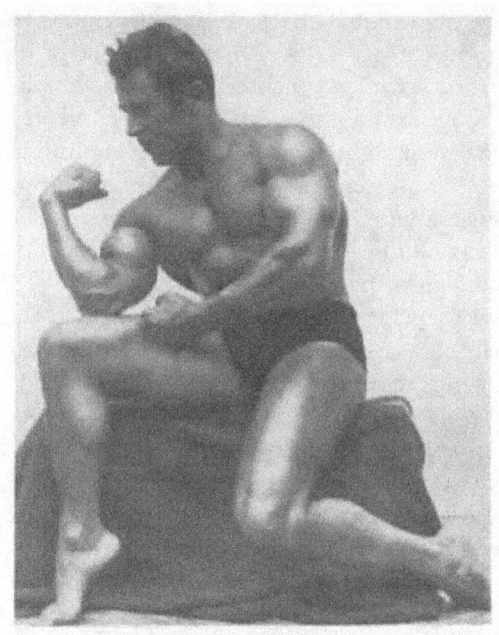

SAM LOPRINZI won the Most Muscular Man title in U.S.A.
in 1946. His 18 inch biceps are notable for their high bulge.
He operates a gymnasium in Portland, Oregon, and is a most
sincere bodybuilder.

There are several systems worth consideration. The
older school of thought has little use for any sort of
specialization to build big arms. They practice a
routine of some dozen exercises for the entire body
and limbs and let the arms come out as they will.
Their chief logic consists of saying that you must
use the arms to hold the barbell or dumb-bell while
doing other exercises, so the arms naturally get
more than their share of exercise. If one followed

this system, the arms might grow to fifteen, or even 16 inches, but you would never get the sort of arms that bodybuilders desire in this day and age.

Other musclemen, the sworn protagonists of Lumps, go all out for a number of highly concentrated and specialized routines. There is the Set System; the SuperSet System, the Peak Concentration System, the Rest- Pause System, the Heavy and Light System, the Multiple Set System, etc., etc. Some are simple systems, using many sets of one or two exercises, and others are in favour of a thousand-and-one different exercises. We might put down right here our own reactions to these various methods. We have observed that men who use a very simple system of perhaps two or three exercises —the curl, the press, and perhaps press on bench—and do many sets of these movements, do get big arms in many cases, but their arms are merely bulky, not shapely. And, on the other hand, the ones who employ a great number of movements over hours of exercise time, are apt to get a high degree of separation and distended blood vessels, and not enough actual bulk and comparable strength. The safe way to go in this, as in almost every human endeavour, is somewhere in the middle of the road.

Thirty-odd years ago, in the first training quarters we had established in our local YMCA, over the vehement protests of the physical director, who swore we would get musclebound, we had a group of lads training with us. At that time we did a routine of some dozen general exercises, and then practised some bent presses, and maybe one or two other lifts. The rest of the gang followed our lead, except for one fellow named Bill. Bill didn't like the agony of doing deep knee bends, and rowing movements and snatches and jerks and bent presses. He did just two exercises—two hand presses and two hand curls. He would repeat these time after time, while the rest of us were doing all-round stuff. I suppose he might have done twenty or thirty sets of presses and curls during an evening. After a few months of this we noticed something. Bill had the biggest upper arms of us all. True, he couldn't snatch anything, and he was no good at cleaning a heavy weight to his shoulders, and he couldn't squat with nearly as much as the rest of us, and he was a sort of an awkward chap, but one day we put the tape on him and found he had sixteen-and-a-half- inch biceps. The " Set " system had been born. The last time I saw Bill, some ten years ago, he still had big arms, but the rest of his physique was nothing to write home about. And, in spite of his curling and pressing, over the years, his arms were not nearly as shapely as they might have been. Further, they never got over a limit of seventeen inches. The Set system, in its simplified form, had worked fairly well, but it was not perfect.

Another time, some twenty years ago, we were greatly interested in weight-lifting, and we had a pretty good team of young fellows at this same

YMCA. Most of our practice, after a starting period of a few months, when general exercises were used, was devoted to doing the three Olympic lifts. A couple of the boys wanted to get bigger arms, so they could walk around town in the summer months with their sleeves rolled up and impress the babes. So, as a concession, we advised them to do just one exercise in addition to their lifting-practice. This was the Dumb-bell Circle movement, done with a pair of twenty-pound dumb-bells. At the close of training, we would all do three sets of just as many reps, as we could squeeze out on this one. Lo and Behold! The whole team got sixteen or better arms! And this, on just one exercise, with a minimum of weight.

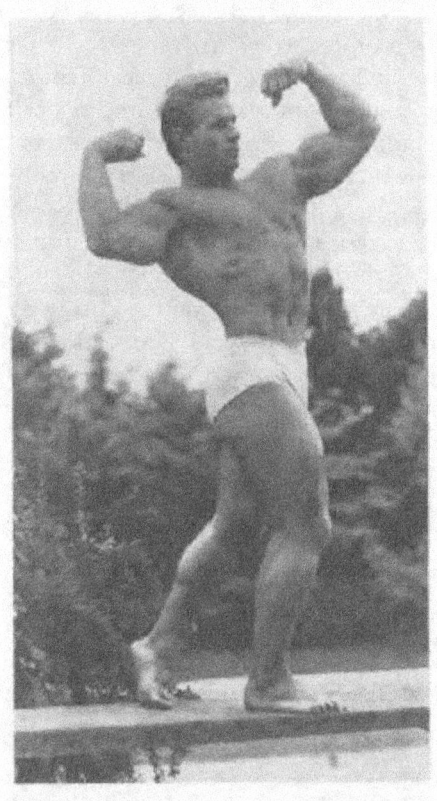

JACK DELINGER, Mr. America, 1949, has a beautifully proportioned physique. His arms, though large, fit perfectly into the overall picture. His physique was built by very heavy workouts; a fact anybody could guess by a glance at this photograph.

Some dozen years ago, we spent quite a lot of time around the York Barbell Club Gym in York, Pennsylvania. Probably the most famous strength and muscle stars in the whole world trained at York.

Back around 1940 a big six-footer from the neighbouring village of Carlisle named Jake Hitchens began to haunt the gym. Jake was not at all interested in strength, but he was enthralled by huge muscular girths. He had the idea that the way to get big muscles was to do exercises with big weights. So he followed John Grimek and Steve Stanko through their exercise routines, but instead of using 25-lb. to 60-lb. dumb-bells in the various chest-and shoulder-building routines used by these mighty champions, he insisted on using 75-lb. and 100-lb. dumb-bells. Of course, he couldn't do the movements exactly like John and Steve, so he bent his arms at the elbow instead of keeping the arms straight, and thus reduced the strain. He did curls by bouncing, bending back, and swinging the bell; he pressed the bar overhead with a push and shove. He absolutely refused to do deep knee bends. Results: Jake grew 18-inch arms and a 50-inch chest. He was the first man, to our knowledge, to go all-out for " Cheating ' exercises.

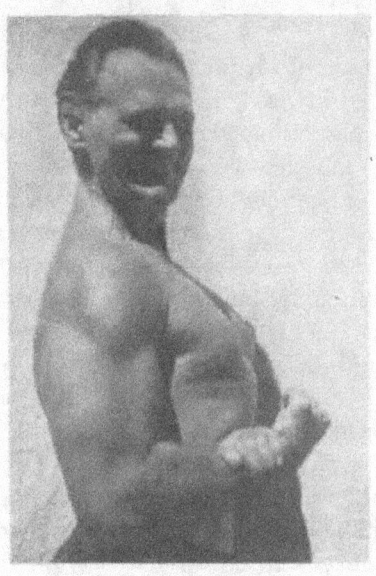

ROBERT W. NEALEY, of Greenwich, Conn., is a well-known American author (mystery, sports, westerns), who was for many years a lifting champion in New England. Now past forty, he has built the impressive (near 17 inch) arms shown in this photo through practice of the exercises listed in this book. (He is also one of the author's best friends and severest critics!)

We would like to say, at this point, that Jake got very strong from this unorthodox practice, but this would not be so. He got bulk, it is true, but he was never anyway near as strong as he looked. We recall one time when the York boys played a dirty trick on Hitchens. There were four lifting platforms in the big gym, and each of them had a revolving York International bar. Jake liked to use the one on a platform close to the Dream Bench, so he could sit down and relax. (The Dream Bench was so-called because so many lifters had rested on it while dreaming of becoming World Champion.) This bar, like the others, was usually loaded-up with a pair of 45-lb. discs, which, with the 45-lb. weight of the bar, made up a barbell with a weight of 135 lb. (minus collars). Jake was accustomed to seizing this bar and doing a set of perhaps ten rough, violent presses to start his workout. Unknown to Hitchens, and to other strangers as well, the boys at the York foundry had cast a number of plates somewhat thicker than the regular 45-lb. discs, which looked exactly like the usual weights. These super-discs weighed 75 lb. So one day the boys fixed up Jake's favourite bar with seventy-fives instead of forty-fives, so that it weighed 195 lb. instead of 135.

Jake, always a breezy conversationalist, came rushing into the gym, full of vim, vigour and vitality. He felt super, he opined, and would show the boys how to take a real rough workout. He grabbed his warm-up bell. It went to the shoulders, a little harder than usual, but when he started to push it vigorously overhead, his first violent shove only carried it as high as his nose, and it began to sink downward. The boys in the gym began to gather round. " What's the trouble, Jake? " they asked solicitously. "Are you sick? Do the weights feel heavy to-day? " Poor Jake was completely dumbfounded. He thought he was losing his strength. He tried the bar again, and again, and still couldn't lift it. He asked one of the others to try it, and of course the weight of 195 meant nothing to guys like Grimek and Stanko, and they played with it like a toy. Poor Hitchens decided he should see a doctor, and reluctantly put on his street clothes and went away. The next time he came into the gym the 75-lb. phoney plates had been removed, and Jake was back to normal.

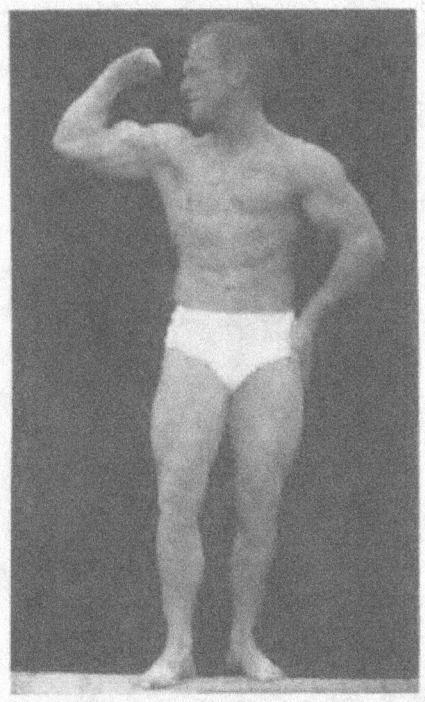

ELLWOOD HOLBROOK typifies the rugged man of muscle. A long-time lifting champion, he has also won honours in the physique field. He has bent-pressed 278½ lbs. with one hand; military pressed 235, snatched 235, jerk 305 lbs. He is 5 feet, 7 inches, weighs 175 lbs. The arm is 16 inches, and it is not bad, is it?

The boys at York did a lot of experimentation with all sorts of odd equipment and gym furniture. They rigged up several pulleys, and were among the first to do pulley or " Lat " machine exercises. They also had built very crudely, the first Incline Bench I ever saw. This bench had a seat about half-way up the incline, and was consequently very comfortable to use. Stanko, Grimek, Bacon, Lauriano and others, spent most of their exercise time upon this piece of furniture, using dumb-bells of varying weights. The flat bench was seldom used, except by Stanko, who liked to pull over bars in excess of 300 lb. over his head from the floor, and then do a press or two. I have never seen Grimek on the flat bench, which may explain the normal beauty of his flat, athletic, pectoral muscles, so much in contrast with the other over-pecced musclemen of this era, whose fondness for bench-presses has " done them wrong."

You can travel the world over and not find better arms than those of Grimek and Stanko, whose biceps tape from 18½ to 19 inches. Dumb-bell exercises on the incline bench were responsible for the finishing touches on these arms. Before they ever did any incline bench movements, they had big, strong arms from their practice as champion weightlifters, but their arms were not so rounded and shapely. We must conclude, therefore, that dumb-bell exercises of this type have a very beneficial effect in shaping super-arms.

About five years previous to this particular period another York barbell man was distinguished for unusual arm-development. He was Dave Mayor, the York heavyweight between the Bill Good period and Stanko's time. Dave was really a bodybuilder rather than a lifter, and before he came to York had done all his exercising in the family kitchen in Philadelphia. He was about 6' 3" tall, and weighed about 250 lb. To him must be attributed the discovery of the value of developing the brachialis as a contribution to biceps size. Dave's favourite movements were barbell exercises; the pull-up to chin, and the rowing movement with weights over 300 lb. He got arms over 19 inches around in the day when 17-inch arms were considered extraordinary. I can remember the incredulous look on Sig Klein's face when he told me in Philly, " Did you feel that guy's arms? I thought they would be like mush—and they are hard as iron! " When Dave stood on the lifting-platform, all one could see was those huge bulging arms.

At this same period, a light-heavy named Steve Gob, of New Jersey, was competing in American lifting, and finishing right up at the top. He pressed 270 lb. in a perfect military press back before 1940. He had a pair of the finest arms and shoulders we have ever seen, and we inquired about them. It seemed that in the Jersey Gym he frequented, the boys had a habit of competing on lifting heavy dumb-bells, doing alternate presses, and also pressing them simultaneously. He did a lot of see-saw presses with a pair of hundreds, and had succeeded with hundred-and-twenty-fives. All of the men in this gym had remarkable arms and shoulders. Later on, Stan Stanczyk devoted a lot of time to dumb-bell presses, and his Olympic press went up from 230 to nearly 300 lb. Over the years, we have found no better exercise for the arms and shoulders combined than dumb-bell pressing of this type. Sig Klein had used this to great advantage back around 1925 in building the best physique of his era. He once did ten reps (each arm) with a pair of hundreds.

It is significant that Louis Uni (Apollon) used to use blockweights in his act, gripping several of these awkward weights together, and doing swings and snatches with them. His magnificently shaped 20-in. arms testify to the effectiveness of single-armed movements with dumb-bells.

We trained in the same gym, with Johnny McWilliams, who has probably the largest arms of to-day (they run from 20 to 21 inches), and with Eric Pedersen, who was runner-up to Steve Reeves for " Mr. America " 1947, and who had the highest hump on the biceps we ever saw, and 18-inch arms as well. We learned something from each of these men. From McWilliams, the value of the French Press, or Triceps Curl; and from Pedersen the shaping value of the " cramp " curl, or peak contraction curling.

Peary Rader, editor of Iron Man Magazine, once used a rather unique form of rest-pause arm training, which he said put a full inch on his arms in two weeks. ' Being in a gymnasium all day long, he was able to use this system, which would be impractical to the average man. He started in the morning and did two exercises only, one for biceps, one for triceps, using about ten reps, on each. He did a curl for the biceps, and a French Curl for the triceps. He would do two sets of ten reps, each on each of these movements, thus working both triceps and biceps pretty thoroughly, but not to exhaustion. Then he would take a full hour's rest while he did other work. At that time he would repeat his two exercises another two sets. Then another hour's rest. He did this throughout the day—usually doing six exercise sessions.

He also did a little muscle " cramping " after each session, to be sure the muscle was thoroughly flooded with blood. This is somewhat similar to the system used by many weightlifters to increase their poundage in the press. This is a good " blitz " technique, but cannot be pursued for more than a couple of weeks at a time, or you will find yourself all washed up. Any time you try to do daily exercise you will come pretty shortly to a sticking point, and the only thing to do is rest for a week.

We have come to certain well-shaped conclusions about barbell training after many years in the game. We think many prominent body culturists of the present day have demonstrated their training ideas are wrong by the misshapen condition of their bodies. The period of endless sets (one exercise repeated ad infinitum) has had its heyday and is definitely over. All that anyone may expect from limited use of a muscle is unbalanced over-development. The arms must be worked from a number of angles to make a fully developed, balanced arm. We think, too (as we have always thought), that an arm must be strong in order to look strong. The use of " cramping " lightweight exercises should not be overdone. Yet we also feel, conversely, that many weightlifters would have better arms if they did include the practice of some shaping or muscle-moulding exercises as well as their pure strength movements.

In the schedules of exercises which we set up in another chapter, you will find that all of these contain a strength- building exercise, followed by a muscle-moulding movement. We believe this is the way to the perfect arm.

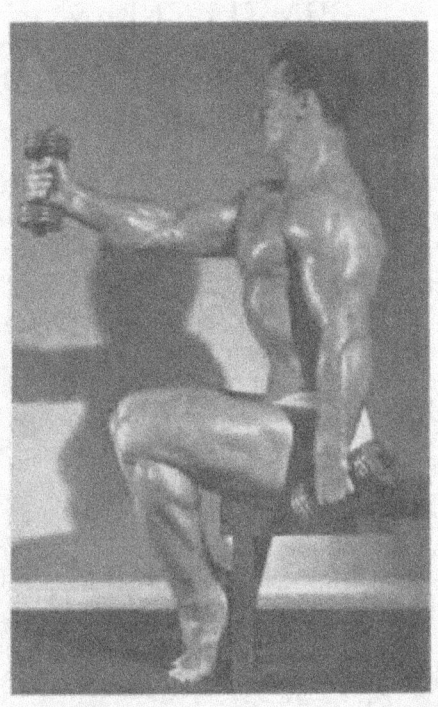

This photo of the incomparable GRIMEK shows him doing a
deltoid exercise, seated. The perfection of the Grimek
shoulders is a result of many dumb-bell movements with com-
paratively light weights.

CHAPTER THREE

EXERCISES FOR THE ARMS AND SHOULDERS

EXERCISE 1.—One of the oldest of all exercise movements is CHINNING THE BAR. There are many variations of this; using a palms-in or palms-out grip, variations in width of handgrip, gripping the wrist, forearm or upper arm of one hand with the other, finally leading to the one-hand chin. We put this exercise first, not because it is the best biceps developer, but because it is so well known. What boy hasn't tried to see how many times he could chin, in contests with his playmates? It is also a non-apparatus movement and can be practised by anyone \yho finds barbells and dumb-bells unavailable. The movement itself is simple. You simply hang at full- length and pull the body upward until the chin is above the bar. The wide-arm chin, pulling the body up until the back of the neck touches the bar is a great favourite with some of our best known bodybuilders. It affects the latissimus more than the arms. The bar should be gripped with palms toward the body for better biceps results.

EXERCISE 2.—The PUSH-UP is the second well-known movement practised by almost everyone. This is the standard non-apparatus triceps developer. It may be made progressive by starting with the simple movement on the floor, then

38

between chairbacks or on parallel bars, then elevations of the feet until finally push-ups are done in the handstand position. This exercise, particularly handstand push-ups, tiger bends, etc., is a favourite of the very best physique stars. One of the advantages of these first two exercises is that after you have developed powerfully-muscled arms you can keep them in good condition by doing chins and push-ups when apparatus is not available.

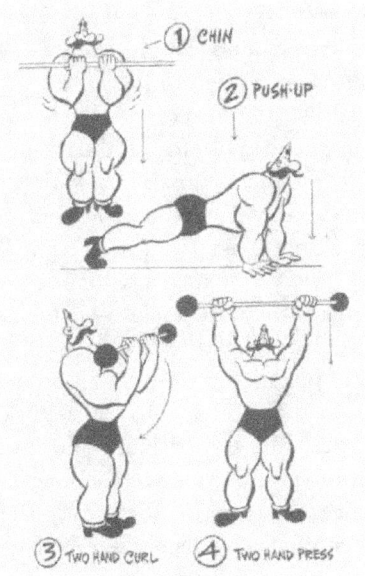

EXERCISE 3.—The TWO-HAND CURL is the number- one barbell exercise for the biceps. You grasp the bar with the undergrip (palms forward) about shoulder-width apart. The arms are held

straight, you breathe in deeply and bring the hands up until the arms are fully flexed. The elbows come forward slightly at the end of the movement, to facilitate flexion. Turning the wrists in to start the curl helps to flex the biceps. Breathe out as you lower the bar to full arm's length in front of the thighs. Be sure to forcibly straighten the arms, until you feel the triceps " lock-out " at the bottom of each curl.

EXERCISE 4.—The TWO-HAND PRESS is essentially a triceps and deltoid exercise. The bar is grasped with the overgrip, slightly more than shoulder-width apart. You pull it in to the shoulders by squatting before the bar, toes under it, feet six or eight inches apart, back flat. The arms are loose, and the pull starts slowly, then accelerates as the bar comes past the knees. The knees are dipped slightly as you turn the hands over at the shoulders, then they are locked stiffly before you begin to press overhead. Locking the hip section, swaying the pelvis forward is recommended, in order to get a firm base to press upon. Now, breathing in deeply, the barbell is pushed to arm's length, keeping it in as close to the face as possible. As it reaches the top of the head, the press is slightly backward to secure an easy armlock. Breathe out as the bell is lowered to the chest or collarbone, upon which the bar should rest to start the movement. Do not rest a press upon the raised deltoids to start.

EXERCISE 5.—The SWINGBAR CURL is a newer exercise, a favourite of John Grimek and Steve Stanko. A short thirteen-inch bar is used, with the discs in the centre, so the hands may grip outside the weight. It is performed in a seated position, with the torso bent forward, the thighs spread so the bar may descend between the legs. The bell is curled right in to the neck, permitting a very complete flexion of the biceps, and when lowered, the triceps are locked out forcibly at the bottom of the arc. This makes the swingbar curl an almost ideal muscle-moulding exercise for the entire arm. The hands are close together, which intensifies the "cramping" action at the top of the curl.

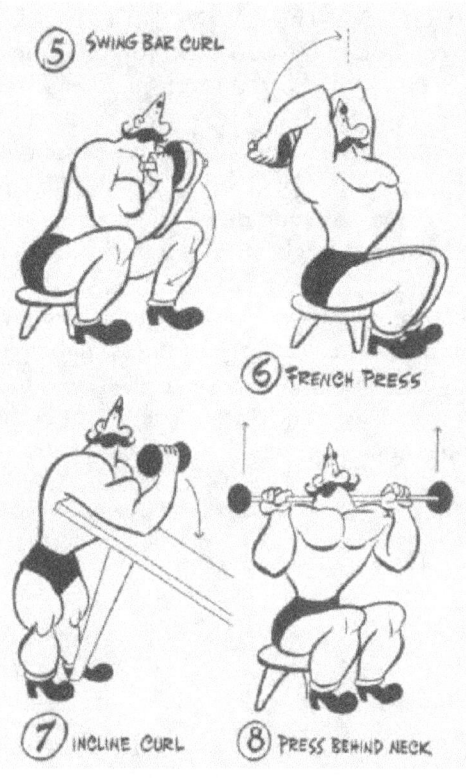

EXERCISE 6.—The FRENCH PRESS, also erroneously called a " triceps curl ", affects the triceps in the same sort of a high contraction manner as you get for the biceps in the preceding exercise. This makes it exceedingly valuable as a muscle-moulder or shaping exercise. The swingbell may also be used very well here, although a barbell is satisfactory. This is best done seated, the bar is

first held straight overhead, then lowered to the back of neck, while keeping the elbows stationary. This is important—the elbows must remain pointing straight up, only the forearms move. This may also be done while lying on a bench, with slightly different effect.

EXERCISE 7.—The INCLINE CURL is another of the muscle-moulding movements. This is done by standing at the head of an incline bench (45 degree angle), and extending the whole arm down the bench, so that it rests against the bench along its whole length. The dumb-bell is now curled in to the shoulder, without lifting any portion of the upper arm from contact. You must not lift the shoulder.

EXERCISE 8.—The PRESS BEHIND NECK has an even better concentrated effect on both triceps and deltoids than the regular standing two-hand press. Many now prefer to do this movement while seated, but that position is optional. The barbell is first " cleaned " to the shoulders, then tossed overhead to rest up on the back of the shoulders. The hands must of necessity take a wide grip, which naturally places more work on the shoulder muscles. The head is leaned forward, and the weight pressed to arm's length. As the bell passes the top of the head, it comes forward slightly, just as the bar goes slightly backward in the regular press. In all these exercises, breathe in fully and deeply as the bar moves up, and breathe out strongly as the bar comes down.

EXERCISE 9.—DUMB-BELL CURLS on Incline Bench are splendid muscle-moulders. The use of dumb-bells allows greater flexibility of movement, and full flexion and extension may be secured. The position also keeps body-motion out of the exercise, insuring that all work is done by the arm muscles. The fact that the arms hang slightly backwards because of gravity helps to make this ideal for locking out the triceps at the bottom of the arc. Lift the elbows at the finish of the curl to intensify the " cramp " effect on biceps.

EXERCISE 10.—The TRICEPS RAISE behind back with barbell is another wonderful muscle-moulding movement. In this the bar is grasped with wide grip, palms forward. From a standing position, with bar held touching the back of the thighs, you keep arms stiff and raise bell upward, at the same time inclining the torso forward until it reaches a position parallel to the floor. You raise the bar just as far as it will go, and then give a little extra lift at the end, to fully knot the inner head of the triceps. This is " muscle-spinning " pure and simple, but it does add to shape and size of the triceps, resulting in a pronounced horseshoe conformation. You may find dumb-bells better in this exercise.

EXERCISE 11—The CRAMP CURL is another pure muscle-spinner. It has been used to give the " lump " on a lump effect to the biceps of many noted physique contestants—notably Eric Pedersen, whom we have seen use it until we thought he would fall flat on his face. It has value as a shaping movement only and is not recommended to pure-strength athletes. This is done either standing or seated, and with the torso bent forward. Pedersen stood and rested his non-lifting hand on some support. The dumb-bell is curled up and slightly inward, to the centre of the neck. The first movements are full extensions, and then the arc is shortened until only halfcurls are made, thus keeping the biceps in a constant state of contraction, until finally the biceps is cramped so tightly it hurts. This is the movement many musclemen refer to when they say they are " pumping up " their arms.

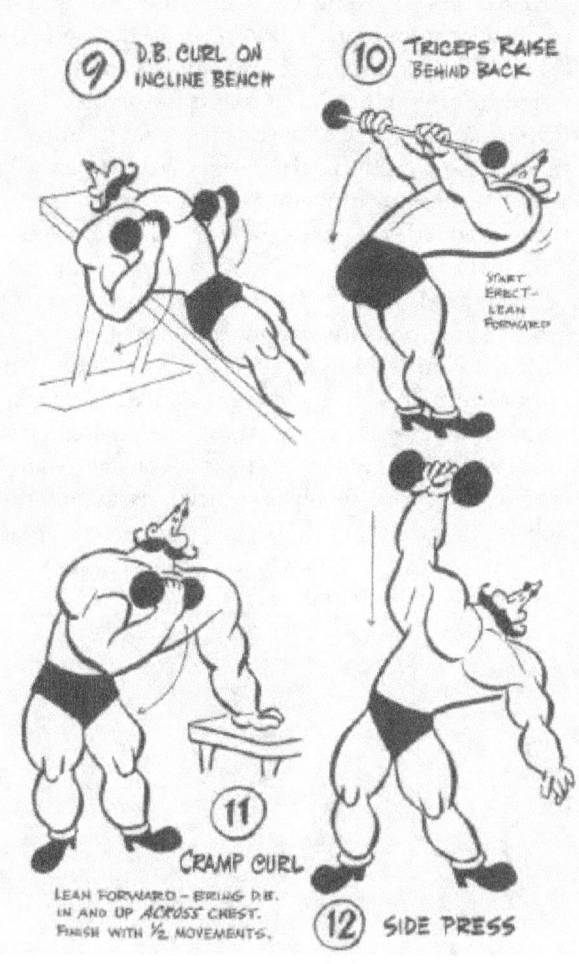

EXERCISE 12.—The ONE-HAND PRESS with dumbbell or barbell was responsible for the

splendid arms of many old-timers, and has unfortunately fallen into disuse in later years. It is a good exercise because it permits a freer and more complete movement of the arm than when two hands are used simultaneously, and it is also inspiring to the trainee because he can flatter his ego by using more weight. It should be done without bending completely over, but with a generous side movement, keeping the legs straight. If the elbow is kept well back on the side to start more weight may be handled, and the developmental effect is also improved.

EXERCISE 13.—The PULLOVER AND PRESS ON BENCH is a good exercise for the triceps, front of deltoids and pectoral muscles. It should not be confused with the currently popular bench press in which the bar is handed to the lifter. We do not approve of this latter exercise because its excessive use has brought about a very unpleasing over development of the pectoral muscles, tending to feminize the male physique. The pullover and press limits the amount of weight handled to the amount the lifter may pull over to the chest, and this part of the exercise is the most important portion.

EXERCISE 14.—One of our personal favourite arm movements is DUMB-BELL CIRCLES, adapted from the old " Zottman " exercise. This is one of the very best muscle- moulders because its action fits perfectly the real function of the biceps.

It builds wrists, forearms, at the same time it affects biceps, triceps and brachialis. The dumbbells alternately describe full flat circles in front of the body, the wrists being turned up at the bottom on the outward arc, and turned downward on the inner arc This exercise alone built a whole class of sixteen-inch arms, or larger, in one of our classes twenty years ago, when no other arm specialization was used by any of the members.

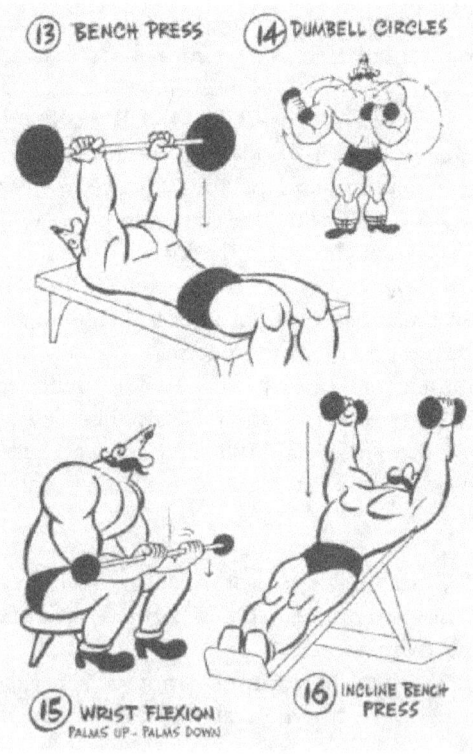

EXERCISE 15.—WRIST FLEXION with forearms supported upon the knees is a good accessory exercise to help develop forearms and wrists proportionate to upper arms. This movement is done with palms turned up and palms turned down. The barbell is usually used, although dumb-bells will probably give wider range of movement, and also permit turning the wrists in a clockwise or counter-clockwise direction.

EXERCISE 16.—The INCLINE BENCH PRESS with dumb-bells is a better developer than the ordinary bench or supine press with barbell. This affects the pectorals and deltoids in a better fashion than the bench press, and gives the high chest, so much admired. Both John Grimek and Steve Stanko owe much of their splendid development to use of dumb-bells on the incline (45 degrees) bench. They do not use extremely heavy weights either. The use of extremely heavy weights in the bench press has been responsible for a great deal of pectoral distortion. You will do better to keep the weight of the dumb-bells to less than 100 lb.

EXERCISE 17.—The PULL-UP to chin with barbell is one of the best deltoid and brachialis exercises known. Use a close grip (about six or eight inches between the hands), stand erect and pull up steadily and strongly until the centre of bar touches the chin. It is said that Herman Goerner could do 286 lb. in this movement. We have seen a number of very strong men do 200 lb. Actually, we would say, the weight used should come somewhere between that which you can curl and the weight you can press. This is one of the MUST exercises on our schedule.

EXERCISE 18.—DELTOID DUMB-BELL EXERCISE is a compound movement. Keeping the arms straight, bells are first lifted to shoulder height from the front, then from the sides. This affects the shoulders from both front and side and helps to round them. Fairly light weights must be used, for this is not a feat of strength, but a muscle-moulding movement. One of Grimek's favourite exercises is to do alternate raises all the way over head, sometimes with palms up, sometimes with palms down and sometimes with palms sideways.

EXERCISE 19.—DUMBELL PRESSES, done alternately (see-saw press) or together, are probably the very best all-round shoulder and arm exercise. Every great strength athlete I have known has done a great deal of dumb-bell work. One hint may help you in handling more weight in either style: try to keep the elbows well back instead of in front of the body. In the alternate press, some body motion, from side to side* helps to start the bells; but this should not be exaggerated, because so doing takes the work from arms and shoulders where it belongs if you are to derive the most benefit from this splendid exercise.

EXERCISE 20.—The WRIST ROLLER is a simple but effective forearm, wrist and finger developer. A round bit of wood, or pipe, about two inches in diameter is ideal for this. Bore a hole through the centre of this bar, place a stout cord through it about three and a-half feet long, and attach a disc to the bottom. Then wind the weight up with arms extended at shoulder height. Turn toward the body—then turn away from the body. Two trips each way will usually leave you with arms paralyzed, if you have attached the proper amount of weight.

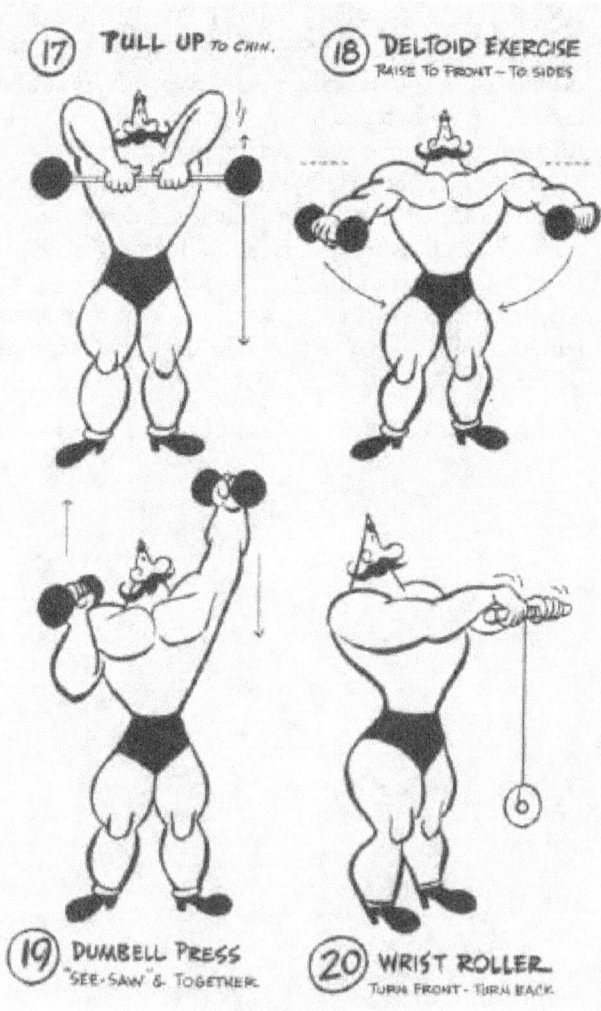

17 PULL UP TO CHIN.

18 DELTOID EXERCISE
RAISE TO FRONT — TO SIDES

19 DUMBELL PRESS
"SEE-SAW" & TOGETHER

20 WRIST ROLLER
TURN FRONT - TURN BACK

CHAPTER FOUR

How TO DO IT - A PROGRAMME FOR ACTION

IN THE preceding chapter we have shown you, mostly through simple illustrations, the best arm and shoulder specialization exercises. One might think the best way to get powerful arms would be to make up a schedule of these twenty movements and go through them daily. Nothing would be further from the truth. Men with perfect arms have learned that too many exercises are just as harmful as too few. And daily exertion is not the way to solid development.

It is true that many top physique stars have used hard daily workouts for a couple of weeks preceding a contest to gain muscular separation, but just as many more have found that this arduous daily toil results in staleness, lack of tone, and even smaller measurements. You will find the daily exercise boys among those who are synthetic strong men; fellows who simply MUST work out every day because they fear that a lost workout will result in a loss of a quarter inch on their biceps. The pure " muscle-spinners " are in this class. Solid musclemen, like Grimek, need only one or two workouts a week to maintain full size and contour.

This is not to say that there is not a place in a specialization programme for daily workouts.

Sometimes a short "Blitz" schedule may make use of a few exercises and daily work, but over the long pull, the best results will come from thrice-a-week workouts. Through tests with many pupils, we have also come to the conclusion that full rest periods about every six weeks are very helpful to continuous progress. There is no profit in going " stale ".

We believe that it takes real hard work to build big arms, but we also see no good reason for becoming slaves to exercise. Three- and four-hour workouts are all right for professionals, but the average chap has to work for a living, and he has only so much energy. Weight- training will add to this energy quotient if properly used. If abused, it cannot fail to do harm instead of good. We conclude that six hours per week is enough exercise for the average man, and is sufficient to give him physical perfection. So our schedules will be based on three two- hour workouts weekly, with at least one day's rest between each session.

Another thing: A great many fellows rush headlong into certain specialization programmes without thought to the body as a whole. Thus, they defeat their purpose. There must be harmonious growth of the whole physique, and unless certain basic exercises are included in even a limited schedule, the results will not be worthwhile. We always include one powerful overall exercise in any specialization programme—usually the breathing squat. And we also include some chest-shaping exercises in between our arm routines. The best breathing exercise we know is the one given first in our book Muscle Moulding, which is done without weight resistance.

Several pupils have told us, upon following this type of arm specialization, that their chests have grown several inches, much to their surprise. That is the very reason we include such movements. You cannot get big-arms without getting a big chest, too. The two go together like fish and chips. The best thing about using a good rousing set of squats at the start of an arm programme is its effect upon the whole bodily metabolism. The body knows it has been working, and demands nourishment for growth. It makes better use of the food you eat, and the arm and shoulder exercises you do in addition to the squat, thus find Mother Nature in a good mood to promote growth.

Another reason many pupils fail to get the desired results from specialized training is because they fail to make use of weight training's most important principle—that of gradual progression. Too many think they merely need to do four, five, or six sets of ten repetitions each of the curl or press, and presto—eighteen-inch arms! They try to force the muscles instead of coaxing them. In our own workouts we have always tried to give interest to training by making each succeeding session a little harder than the last. Sometimes we are only able to squeeze out one more repetition on a certain movement —perhaps we are able to add five pounds to the bar— but always we try to show progress. The effect of this on the mind is important, for the mental side of this muscle-building business is just as productive as the physical. When using this progressive principle you will naturally come to a point where more weight and more reps, are manifestly impractical, and it is then when you should stop and rest for a week and then begin with a different schedule and with somewhat reduced weights.

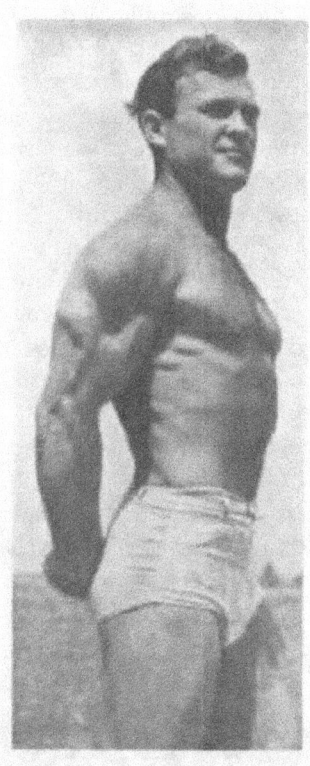

Have you ever seen better triceps than ELLWOOD HOLBROOK shows in this picture. This is the arm that presses 278 lbs., and, mind you, it is not over 16 inches !

In shaping the muscles, we must not overlook the value of muscle control. The Greats of the game have been men who devoted a lot of time to mental massage of the muscle groups. Sandow, Grimek, Klein, Park, and all the other outstanding stars have learned to flex, flick and ripple every

57

muscle band in the arm simply by thinking about it. This mental control has a very beneficial effect on the very shape of the muscles. The biceps themselves learn to leap higher at the word of command. 'It is well to rest the arms between exercises by flexing them, waving them loosely, making the muscles ebb and flow. You can also add to the effectiveness of certain " cramp " movements by exerting this mental control to fully flex the muscle while using a weight. Old-timers like Max Sick and Otto Arco carried this mental control to such peaks of efficiency that their arms were tremendous when measured in the flexed position. Arco had 17-in. biceps when weighing about 140 lb. A point worth remembering, however, is that these short men had superlative allround development, without a single weak link in the chain. They were just as strong as they looked.

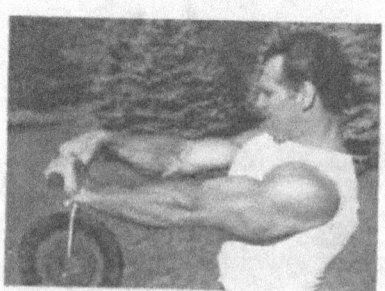

Mighty JOHN GRIMEK doing the wrist roller exercise with a 25 lb. weight. Most men will find 5 to 10 lbs. plenty, but *The Glow* laughs at 25 lbs. What an arm !

It is beneficial, too, to apply physical massage to the muscles after you use them vigorously. Between exercises, rub, knead and gently pinch the muscles you have been using. This helps to loosen them, allows the fatigue poisons to be carried away, and keeps the blood flowing. When using the set system, this is not only beneficial, it is almost imperative if the muscles are to be able to do their three sets without complete fatigue.

If you have ever had occasion to watch a celebrated muscleman in action, you may have noticed how often he rests. Indeed, in a two-hour workout, the Star spends a good three-quarters of the time lounging around. He will do one set of ten curls, for example, then he will do some deep breathing, sit down, relax, perhaps even lie down for perhaps two or three minutes. Then he approaches the bar and does another set. He rests again before doing the final set. It may take him 30 seconds to do 10 reps—and he will rest at least 120 seconds between sets. He does this with all his exercises. This is the best way for the average man to approach his training. Don't rush through it. Work hard when you are actually doing an exercise, and give it all your energy; but always rest long enough between movements to give your heart and lungs time to return to normal. Some people recuperate faster than others. For one, one minute is long enough between sets. For another, three minutes may be desirable. We have found it wise to sprinkle through our own workouts, about ten sessions of forced breathing of from 10 to 20 breaths, holding on to the squat rack and forcing the hands down, as shown in the "Bosco" breathing movement. This has the effect of returning respiration and pulse to normal much faster than if we merely rest, or do nothing. And besides, it is building the chest and getting valuable oxygen into the bloodstream.

Now, let us turn to consideration of actual programmes. The three suggested routines following are intended to be used for six weeks each, with one week of full rest between programmes.

EXERCISE SCHEDULE NO. 1

1.   Warm-up Exercise:
        Do some bends, a couple of squats, Ilex the arms.
2.   Breathing Squats:
        20 Reps. Take 3 deep breaths between last 10.
8.   Bosco Breathing Exercise:
        20 Breaths, pushing down with hands on rack.
4.   Pull-up to Chin.
        5 Reps. Use fairly heavy bar.
5.   Pull-up to Chin:
        10 Reps. Use lighter bar.
6.   Two-hand Press:
        3 Reps. Use heavy bar.
7.   Two-hand Press:

5 Reps. Use lighter bar, and repeat another
set.
8.   Two-hand Curl:
        5 Reps. Use heavy bar.
9.   Two-hand Curl:
        10 Reps. Use lighter bar, and repeat
another set.
10.   Swing Bar Curl:
        12 Reps. Repeat 10 reps, and then 8 reps.
11.   Triceps Raise (Ex. 10):
        12 Reps. Repeat 10 reps, and then 8 reps.
12.   Dumb-bell Deltoid Exercise (Ex. 18):
        Three sets.

EXERCISE SCHEDULE NO. 2

1.   Warm-up Exercise. (As above.)
2.   Breathing Squats. (As above).
3.   Bosco Breathing Exercise. (As Above.)
4.   Pull-up to Chin. (Heavy.)
5.   Pull-up to Chin. (Light.)
6.   Incline-bench DB Press. Three sets; 12, 10
and 8 reps.
7.   French Press. Three sets; 12, 10 and 8 reps.
8.   Incline-bench Curls (Ex. 9). Three sets; 12,
10 and 8 reps.
9.   Cramp Curls (Ex. 11). Three sets; 12, 10
and 8 reps.

10.   Dumb-bell Circles (Ex. 14). Three sets; as many as possible.

11.   Wrist Roller (Ex. 20). Twice each way.

EXERCISE SCHEDULE NO. 3

1.   Warm-up Exercise.

2.   Breathing Squats.

3.   Bosco Breathing Exercise.

4.   Pull-ups. (Heavy and Light.)

5.   Pullover and Press on Bench. (Heavy and Light.) 5 and 10 reps. Two sets;

6.   Dumb-bell Alternate Press (Ex. 19). Three sets; 12, 10 and 8 reps.

7.   Two-hand Curl. (Heavy and Light.) Two sets; 5 and 10 reps.

8.   Dumb-bell Curl on Incline (Ex. 9). Three sets; 12, 10 and 8 reps.

9.   Wrist Flexion (Ex. 15). Two sets palm up; two sets palm down.

10.   Cramp Curl. Three sets.

11.   Triceps Raise (Ex. 10). Three sets.

The amount of weight to use in these exercises must be left to individual selection. But it is important that you keep adding to the weight each week. This means, naturally, that you should start off with a weight quite easy to handle for the full number of sets and reps. Then, each exercise day, try to add a single rep. as you go along, until the beginning of the next week, when you add 1¼ lb. to single-arm exercises, and 1½ lb. to two-hand movements. If you have no discs as small as 1¼ lb., try to keep on making rep. increases for two weeks and add 2½- and 5-lb. weights each fortnight.

After your week of complete rest on the seventh week, begin again with weights very comfortable to handle.